Your Cor
Atrial Fibrillation

A Comprehensive Manual to Treat and
Reverse AFib Quickly and Sustainably

GOODMAN ROBERTS

1

Table Of Contents

CHAPTER ONE

Atrial Fibrillation Simply Explained

How is the Human Heart Constructed and How Does a Healthy Heart Pump?

The human heart has four chambers and four large valves that make sure blood flows in the right direction. The heart starts beating as early as the sixth week of pregnancy.

What is a Normal Heart Rhythm and What Role Does It Play in Health?

A normal heart rhythm, called sinus rhythm, means the atria contract first, followed by the ventricles. This rhythm keeps the heart and the whole body working well. It's crucial for oxygen-rich blood to be pumped from the heart to the organs so they can function properly.

What is Heart Rate and What Does It Indicate?

Heart rate is the number of times the heart beats per minute. A normal resting heart rate is between 50 and 100 beats per minute. During exercise, the heart rate in young people can go up to 190 beats per minute.

What is Atrial Fibrillation and Where Does It Occur?

Atrial fibrillation (AFib) is the most common irregular heart rhythm. It mainly occurs in the left atrium due to extra beats that come from the pulmonary veins.

What Happens in the Heart During Atrial Fibrillation?

In AFib, extra beats create electrical chaos in the atrium, causing an irregular and inefficient heart action.

How Does the Heart Pump During Atrial Fibrillation Compared to a Healthy Heart?

In sinus rhythm, the heart beats rhythmically and efficiently. In AFib, the heart beats irregularly and inefficiently, which can cause symptoms.

What Consequences Can Atrial Fibrillation Have for Your Health?

AFib is common and usually well-tolerated. However, it can lead to strokes. Detecting AFib early is important to prevent strokes and possible death.

Is Atrial Fibrillation a Progressive Disease?

AFib often starts with short episodes that may not be noticeable. Over time, these episodes can become longer and may not stop on their own, leading to persistent AFib.

What is Heart Failure and Why Can Both Diseases Promote Each Other?

Heart failure is a weakness of the heart. Patients with heart failure often develop AFib, and sometimes AFib can lead to heart failure.

CHAPTER TWO

Causes of Atrial Fibrillation

How Common is Atrial Fibrillation in the Population?
AFib is the most common heart rhythm problem, affecting 2.5% of the population. The risk of AFib increases with age.

What Factors Promote Atrial Fibrillation?
AFib is often caused by other health conditions such as obesity, diabetes, high blood pressure, a previous heart attack, or kidney disease.

Which Risk Factors for Atrial Fibrillation Can I Influence Myself and How?
You can influence many risk factors for AFib. These include losing weight, controlling blood pressure with help from your doctor, and treating other conditions like diabetes and kidney disease.

What Causes of Atrial Fibrillation Have to Do with the Heart?

AFib can be caused by changes in heart pressure, valve diseases like leaks or narrowings, and diseases of the heart muscle.

Why Can Existing Heart Disease Affect the Risk of Atrial Fibrillation?

Heart diseases like a previous heart attack can stress healthy parts of the heart, causing AFib.

Which Heart Diseases Increase the Risk of Atrial Fibrillation?

Heart diseases such as valve leaks, valve constrictions, heart attacks, and heart failure can increase the risk of AFib.

Which Diseases of Other Organs Can Promote Atrial Fibrillation?

An overactive thyroid, excessive snoring, and kidney disease can promote AFib. It's important to check thyroid function if you have AFib.

Which Medications Can Cause Atrial Fibrillation as an Unwanted Side Effect?

Thyroid hormones can cause AFib if the dosage is too high.

What Other Causes of Atrial Fibrillation Are Known and Can the Cause Always Be Determined?

The exact cause of AFib cannot always be determined. Tests are important to identify potential causes like valve diseases or heart muscle diseases.

CHAPTER THREE

Symptoms and Early Detection of Atrial Fibrillation

Why is it Important to Detect Atrial Fibrillation Early?

Detecting atrial fibrillation (AFib) early is crucial to prevent strokes. If you notice your heart beating irregularly or too fast, see a doctor right away.

How Do I Recognize the First Signs of Atrial Fibrillation?

AFib symptoms can be subtle. Often, it occurs at night and is missed while sleeping. It's important to get an ECG, especially if you experience tiredness, shortness of breath, or a rapid heartbeat during the day.

Are There Any Tools to Detect a Fluttering Heart?

A fast, irregular pulse is a clinical sign of AFib. You can check your pulse by hand or use devices like a blood pressure monitor with arrhythmia detection. If you suspect an irregular, rapid pulse, contact your doctor.

What Are the Symptoms of Atrial Fibrillation?

Common symptoms include:
- Rapid pulse
- Shortness of breath
- Decreased performance

Sometimes, patients also report:
- Sweating
- Nausea
- Dizziness

How Long Can Symptoms Last and Can They Go Away on Their Own?

AFib symptoms usually last as long as the episode itself. There are two forms of AFib:
- Paroxysmal AFib: Stops on its own
- Persistent AFib: Requires medical intervention, such as medication or electrical cardioversion

When Do the Symptoms Typically Occur?

Many patients develop AFib while resting at night, waking up with an irregular and rapid heartbeat. During physical activity, AFib can cause shortness of breath and decreased performance.

What Should I Do if I Feel Atrial Fibrillation?

If your pulse is fast and irregular, make sure your heart rate doesn't get too high. Sometimes medication is needed, so see a doctor. If you develop acute AFib, sit or lie down to avoid dizziness. If AFib doesn't stop, consult a doctor.

What Can I Do to Relieve My Symptoms?

To relieve severe AFib symptoms, you need to stop the arrhythmia. Often, slowing down the heart rate is enough. Work with your doctor to find the right medication.

What Symptoms are Signs of an Emergency and What Should I Do?

Be cautious if you experience dizziness or collapse due to AFib. Don't go to the doctor alone; get help from a paramedic or a relative.

CHAPTER FOUR

Diagnosis of Atrial Fibrillation

How is Atrial Fibrillation Diagnosed and What Tests Can I Expect?
To diagnose atrial fibrillation (AFib), you need an electrocardiogram (ECG). A 12-lead ECG is the standard test and can be done by your general practitioner or internist. Other methods include implanted loop recorders, event recorders, and a 24-hour ECG. Modern smartwatches can also detect AFib reliably.

What Should I Tell My Doctor?
If you think you have AFib, tell your doctor:
- How often episodes happen
- How long they last
- If they stop on their own
- If you need special maneuvers to stop them, like holding your breath

What Questions Will My Doctor Ask and How Can I Prepare?

Your doctor will find it helpful if you keep a rhythm diary. In this diary, note:
- How often episodes occur
- How long they last
- If episodes are linked to certain activities, like sleeping or physical exertion

What is an ECG and How Does the Examination Work?

An ECG is a painless test that records the electrical activity of the heart using electrodes placed on your body. The ECG curve helps doctors identify arrhythmias and other heart diseases.

What Exactly Can Be Seen in an ECG?

An ECG shows the heart's electrical activity graphically, revealing the heart's rhythm, muscle mass, and any acute issues like a heart attack.

What is a Long-term ECG, How Long Does it Last, and Why is This Test Done?

A long-term ECG, usually lasting 24 hours, is used to detect arrhythmias that may not always be present. It can capture arrhythmias that occur at night.

What Does an ECG Result Look Like?

In an ECG showing AFib, you'll see an irregular heart rhythm. The ECG will show the chaotic activity of AFib compared to the regular beats of a healthy sinus rhythm.

What is a Cardiac Ultrasound and How Does This Examination Work?

Cardiac ultrasound is a painless, quick test that lets doctors see the heart in real time. It helps assess heart muscle function and check for valve issues. During the test, you'll lie on your left side, and an ultrasound probe will scan your chest.

What is a Swallowing Ultrasound and How Does This Examination Work?

A swallowing cardiac ultrasound, done under light anesthesia, involves swallowing a probe to assess the heart chambers from the esophagus. This test is important for checking for clots in the atria and examining the heart valves.

How Should I Prepare for These Examinations?

For a standard heart ultrasound, no special preparation is needed. For a swallowing ultrasound, you should fast for at least six hours.

What Does a Cardiac Ultrasound Result Look Like?

In AFib, the ultrasound will show an irregular rhythm and abnormal atrial activity.

CHAPTER FIVE

The Three Types of Atrial Fibrillation: Which One Do You Have?

Atrial fibrillation (AFib) is a type of irregular heartbeat, but there are three different forms of this condition. Each type requires specific treatment, and understanding which one you have can help with your prognosis.

How Do the Three Types of AFib Differ?

The main differences are in the duration and frequency of AFib episodes. This means how long each episode lasts and what needs to be done to stop it.

Paroxysmal AFib: When Problems Come and Go

Paroxysmal AFib is when your heart suddenly starts to beat irregularly and then stops just as suddenly. These episodes can last from a few minutes to a few days and often happen without warning. They can be very noticeable because of the sudden and unpredictable nature of the symptoms, like heart palpitations.

Persistent AFib: When Arrhythmias Persist Without Intervention

Persistent AFib lasts for more than a week and usually needs medication or a procedure called cardioversion to return the heart to a normal rhythm. Cardioversion can be done with medication through an IV or with electrical shocks. Symptoms are similar to those of paroxysmal AFib, including palpitations, rapid heartbeat, dizziness, fatigue, weakness, and shortness of breath. If symptoms are hard to control, a surgical procedure called catheter ablation might be necessary.

Long-lasting Persistent AFib: When the Heart Rhythm Cannot Be Corrected

Long-lasting persistent AFib, also known as permanent AFib, lasts for more than a year and doesn't respond to treatments like medication, cardioversion, or catheter ablation. This type can be very challenging to manage and can lead to constant worry, stress, anxiety, and fatigue, affecting your quality of life.

The Cause Determines the Form

AFib is often a symptom of another condition. Finding the underlying cause can help determine the type of AFib and how it might progress.

- Structural Defect: Problems with heart valves can cause the heart muscle to enlarge, leading to AFib. If you have heart valve disease, you are more likely to develop persistent AFib.
- Secondary AFib: Caused by another condition like a heart attack, sleep apnea, or alcohol abuse. Treating the underlying condition can often reduce or eliminate AFib.
- Primary AFib: When no cause can be found. This might actually be secondary AFib with an unknown cause or occur independently. It can be difficult to treat and often starts with medications before moving to more invasive methods.
- Post-operative AFib: Sometimes AFib occurs after heart surgery due to factors like fluid and electrolyte imbalances or pre-existing conditions. This type can make recovery harder and increase the risk of complications.

The Better You Know Your AFib, the Better You Can Control It

AFib is a progressive disease, meaning paroxysmal AFib can develop into persistent and eventually permanent AFib. The key is to control AFib as soon as possible to improve your health. Monitoring your symptoms closely and communicating with your doctor is essential. Knowledge about your condition can empower you to protect your heart in the future.

CHAPTER SIX

Atrial Fibrillation and Stroke

Understanding Atrial Fibrillation and Stroke
In a healthy heart, electrical signals from the sinus node in the right atrium make the atria contract and pump blood into the ventricles. In atrial fibrillation (AFib), this process is disrupted because many cells try to act as the pacemaker, causing chaotic electrical impulses. This makes the atria quiver instead of contracting properly, and the heart beats irregularly, which is often felt as "heart palpitations."

When the atria fibrillate, blood isn't pumped through the heart correctly. Blood flow slows down, especially in small pockets in the atria called atrial appendages. This can lead to blood clots (thrombi) forming. If a clot breaks off, it can travel to other organs and block an artery, causing an organ infarction, such as a stroke in the brain.

What is a Stroke and How Dangerous is It?

A stroke happens when a blood clot gets stuck in a brain vessel, blocking blood flow. This can cause brain tissue to stop working. Strokes can range from mild, with temporary or slight impairments like hand numbness, to severe or fatal. Symptoms can include needing a wheelchair or being bedridden.

How Do Blood Clots Form and Reach the Brain?

In AFib, blood clots often form in the atrial appendage. These clots can travel through the left ventricle and the main artery to the brain, causing a stroke.

Why is Stroke Risk Higher in People with AFib?

The risk of stroke increases in AFib because blood clots can form in the atrial appendage. If these clots travel to the brain, they can cause a stroke.

Factors Affecting Stroke Risk

The risk of stroke in people with AFib depends on other health conditions and factors like age. For example, an older person with diabetes or a previous stroke has a higher risk than a young, healthy person.

Estimating and Predicting Stroke Risk
Scientists have developed methods to estimate stroke risk accurately. These calculations consider age, other health conditions, and whether a stroke has occurred before.

Preventing Stroke in AFib Patients
Detecting AFib early and starting blood-thinning therapy can greatly reduce the risk of stroke.

Signs of a Stroke
Signs of a stroke can vary widely, including:
- Paralysis, often affecting the face, arm, or one side of the body.
- Speech disorders, making it hard to speak or articulate words properly.

What to Do if You Suspect a Stroke
A stroke is an emergency, similar to a heart attack. Seek medical help immediately. Timely treatment can sometimes reverse the effects of a stroke.

Consequences and Treatment of Stroke

The effects of a stroke can range from minor paralysis to being bedridden or even death. However, treatments like catheter procedures or rehabilitation can help reduce some of the effects.

CHAPTER SEVEN

Dealing with Atrial Fibrillation After Eating

Atrial fibrillation (AFib) is a common heart rhythm disorder that can affect your daily life. By making some conscious changes to your diet and lifestyle, especially around meals, you can help manage AFib symptoms. This doesn't mean giving up tasty food, but understanding how certain foods and habits can affect your heart and adjusting accordingly. Let's explore how to manage AFib after eating.

Key Tips for Managing AFib After Eating

- Identify and Avoid Triggers: Recognize foods and habits that trigger your AFib, such as large meals, alcohol, and caffeine.
- Heart-Healthy Diets: Following a heart-healthy diet like the Mediterranean or plant-based diet can reduce risk factors like high cholesterol and blood pressure.
- Lifestyle Factors: Manage post-meal hypertension with mindful eating, portion control, good sleep, and stress reduction techniques.

How Food Influences AFib Episodes

Everyone with AFib experiences it differently. For some, certain foods can trigger episodes. Common triggers include:

- Large Meals: Eating too much at once can lead to AFib episodes.
- Alcohol: Drinking alcohol, especially more than occasionally, can increase the likelihood of AFib and contribute to heart issues.
- Caffeine: Be aware of caffeine's effects, as it can dehydrate and trigger AFib.

Common Food Triggers

- Fried Foods: Especially when eaten in large quantities, fried foods can trigger AFib.
- Large Meals: Eating large meals can cause AFib.
- Healthy Choices: Including green leafy vegetables in your diet can help prevent AFib by providing essential nutrients and maintaining electrolyte balance.

Personal Sensitivities

Some people may have personal sensitivities to certain foods or substances that can trigger AFib, including:

- Alcohol
- Caffeine
- Gluten
- Red meat
- Processed foods
- Sugary foods and drinks
- Too much salt

An elimination diet can help identify these sensitivities. This involves removing foods that might cause symptoms and then gradually reintroducing them to see if symptoms return.

Why Does Food Cause AFib? The Role of the Vagus Nerve

Eating, especially large meals, can sometimes trigger AFib because of the vagus nerve. The vagus nerve connects the gut, brain, and heart. When you eat, the vagus nerve is stimulated, which can change your heart rhythm and trigger AFib.

The vagus nerve helps control heart rate, so when it's highly activated during digestion, it can cause an irregular heartbeat or AFib. This is why some people experience AFib symptoms after meals.

Managing AFib After Eating

Knowing that food can trigger AFib helps in managing the condition. Eating a balanced diet and avoiding overeating can reduce the risk of triggering AFib after meals. Always aim for a healthy and balanced diet to support your heart health.

A Heart-Healthy Diet for Atrial Fibrillation Treatment

Adopting a heart-healthy diet can greatly help in treating atrial fibrillation (AFib). Diets like the Mediterranean and plant-based diets focus on eating lots of fruits, vegetables, and healthy fats, which can improve heart health and lower cholesterol, reducing the risk of heart attack.

Key Dietary Changes

- Reduce Red Meat: Red meat has more saturated fats than white meat. Eating less red meat can help lower cholesterol levels, which is important for managing AFib.

Mediterranean Diet

The Mediterranean diet is well-known for promoting heart health. It includes a lot of monounsaturated fats from olive oil, which help lower bad cholesterol. This diet can also help reduce risk factors for heart disease, like high cholesterol and high blood pressure.

Research shows that the Mediterranean diet might help prevent or even reverse AFib. People who follow this diet are less likely to develop AFib. It can also improve heart health in those who already have AFib.

Plant-Based Diet

A plant-based diet is another great option for managing AFib. This diet includes:

- Vegetables
- Fruits
- Whole grains
- Legumes
- Non-animal proteins

A plant-based diet not only helps treat AFib but also reduces the risk of heart attack and stroke. With many delicious options, like chickpea pasta with mushrooms and kale or vegan curried vegetables, you can enjoy tasty meals while staying healthy.

Reducing High Blood Pressure After Meals
Mindful Eating

Managing high blood pressure, a risk factor for AFib, is especially important after meals. Mindful eating involves being aware of what and how you eat. This includes:

- Eating slowly
- Paying attention to food
- Choosing lean proteins
- Chewing thoroughly to help digestion

Mindful eating can help control hypertension, which is crucial for managing AFib after eating.

Portion Control

Eating large meals can temporarily raise blood pressure because more blood is needed for digestion. Controlling portion sizes can help manage blood pressure and support a heart-healthy diet.

Alcohol and Atrial Fibrillation

Alcohol can increase the likelihood of AFib episodes. Drinking even one drink per day can raise the risk of AFib by 6%. Chronic alcohol consumption can lead to changes in heart structure and function, worsening AFib.

However, stopping alcohol use can reverse some of these effects. This should be done under medical supervision.

Sleep Apnea and Atrial Fibrillation

Good sleep is vital for overall health, especially for people with AFib. Sleep apnea can change heart function and structure, increasing the risk of AFib. Ensuring regular, restful sleep can significantly reduce this risk compared to those who suffer from insomnia, snoring, and daytime fatigue.

Summary

A heart-healthy diet and lifestyle changes can greatly help manage AFib. By choosing the right foods, controlling portions, avoiding triggers like alcohol, and ensuring good sleep, you can improve your heart health and reduce the risk of AFib episodes.

Stress Management Techniques for Atrial Fibrillation Prevention

Managing stress is important for preventing atrial fibrillation (AFib). Chronic stress and anxiety can trigger AFib episodes, making it crucial to find ways to reduce stress.

Yoga and Mindfulness

- Yoga: Yoga can reduce AFib symptoms, lower stress, and improve quality of life for those with AFib.
- Mindfulness and Deep Breathing: These techniques can help reduce the frequency and severity of AFib by promoting relaxation and addressing emotional triggers.

Caffeine and Energy Drinks: Effects on Atrial Fibrillation

Caffeine and energy drinks can affect AFib in different ways:
- Moderate Caffeine Intake: Some people may find that moderate caffeine consumption reduces the risk of AFib.
- Excessive Caffeine Intake: Too much caffeine can trigger or worsen AFib symptoms. Monitoring your caffeine intake is key to finding what works best for you.

Key Components of the Program

- Dietary Changes: Heart-friendly diet recommendations to avoid AFib triggers.
- Physical Activity: Customized exercise plans based on fitness level and health.
- Stress Management: Techniques like mindfulness, yoga, and breathing exercises.
- Sleep Hygiene: Tips for improving sleep quality to support heart health.

By following this program, individuals can manage AFib and improve overall health and quality of life.

Summary

Managing AFib involves more than just medication. It includes a holistic approach with diet, lifestyle changes, and mindful practices. By making these changes, you can live a healthier and more fulfilling life.

Frequently Asked Questions

Why Does Atrial Fibrillation Start After Eating?

Eating a large meal can stimulate the vagus nerve, which connects the gut, brain, and heart, potentially leading to AFib.

How to Stop Heart Palpitations After Eating?

To avoid heart palpitations after eating, try:

- Reducing portion sizes
- Limiting alcohol consumption
- Drinking plenty of fluids
- Eating regularly
- Monitoring caffeine intake
- Reducing salt and sugar intake

Can Food Affect Atrial Fibrillation?

Certain foods can trigger AFib symptoms. Monitoring your diet and avoiding or limiting certain foods can help manage AFib. Consider a Mediterranean or plant-based diet and reduce saturated fat, salt, and added sugar intake.

What Makes Atrial Fibrillation Worse?

AFib can be worsened by:

- Stress
- Alcohol
- Caffeine
- Certain exercises
- Foods with monosodium glutamate (MSG)

Being aware of these triggers can help you avoid them.

How Can a Mediterranean Diet Help Treat Atrial Fibrillation?

A Mediterranean diet can help manage AFib by addressing heart disease risk factors like high cholesterol and high blood pressure. It supports overall heart health.

CHAPTER EIGHT

Treatments of Atrial Fibrillation

Atrial fibrillation (AFib) requires treatment to reduce the risk of stroke and improve symptoms that affect daily life.

Why Treat Atrial Fibrillation?
- Health Risks: AFib increases the risk of stroke and can lead to other health problems if left untreated.
- Symptoms: Many people with AFib experience symptoms like shortness of breath, rapid heartbeat, or reduced energy.

Urgency of Treatment
- Prompt Attention: New symptoms like heart palpitations should be addressed promptly, though emergency care is rarely needed.
- Medical Attention: Most cases can be managed by seeing a family doctor or specialist within a few days.

Does Everyone Need Treatment?
- Evaluation: If diagnosed with AFib, a thorough evaluation is needed to assess other health

conditions, the need for blood thinners, and create a treatment plan.

Realistic Treatment Goals

- Stroke Prevention: Treatment aims to significantly reduce the risk of stroke by 70 to 80%.
- Improved Quality of Life: Treatment can also enhance quality of life by alleviating symptoms and potentially reducing mortality rates.

Treatment Options

- Medication: Many patients manage AFib with medications that control heart rate (frequency control).
- Procedures: Some patients may require minimally invasive procedures like cardiac catheterization to restore normal heart rhythm (rhythm control).
- Pacemaker: In rare cases, a pacemaker may be needed for patients with very slow heart rates due to AFib.

Frequency Control vs. Rhythm Control

- Frequency Control: Keeps the heart in AFib but manages symptoms by controlling heart rate.

- Rhythm Control: Restores and maintains normal heart rhythm (sinus rhythm) using more invasive methods when necessary.

Choosing the Right Therapy
- Factors to Consider: Age, overall health, symptom severity, and other health conditions influence whether frequency or rhythm control is recommended.
- Personalized Care: The treatment plan should be tailored to each individual's specific needs and health circumstances.

Positive Influence on Disease Course
- Patient's Role: You play a crucial role in managing AFib through lifestyle changes:
  - Healthy Diet: Eat nutritious foods and manage weight.
  - Exercise: Engage in regular endurance activities.
  - Manage Other Conditions: Control diabetes, high blood pressure, and other health issues effectively.

Conclusion
Managing AFib involves understanding treatment options, choosing the right approach based on individual factors, and actively

participating in lifestyle improvements. By working closely with healthcare providers and making healthy choices, you can effectively manage AFib and improve your overall health.

How to Monitor Your Heart Activity at Home

Monitoring your heart activity at home is important for detecting early signs of cardiovascular issues. Here are simple ways to keep track:

1. Measure Blood Pressure:

Regularly check your blood pressure using a blood pressure monitor. High blood pressure can indicate heart problems.

2. Monitor Your Pulse:

Measure your pulse to track your heart rate. This can be done manually by feeling your pulse or using a digital device.

3. Listen to Your Body:

Pay attention to how you feel. Notice if you experience symptoms like racing heart or palpitations, which could indicate conditions like atrial fibrillation.

Using Modern Devices

Modern smartphones and gadgets often have apps or features that can monitor your pulse and heart rhythm. While these can be useful tools, they are not necessary for everyone.

Importance of Regular Medical Check-ups

If you have been diagnosed with atrial fibrillation or any heart condition, regular medical check-ups are crucial:

- Annual Check-ups: Schedule a comprehensive health examination with your doctor at least once a year. This helps monitor your overall health and adjust your treatment plan as needed.

- Additional Visits: Depending on your treatment and medications, you may need more frequent visits. For example, if you are on blood thinners, regular checks of your blood clotting status may be necessary.

Regular check-ups ensure that any changes in your health are detected early, allowing for timely adjustments to your treatment plan. This proactive approach can help manage your condition effectively and improve your quality of life.

Blood Clot Prevention in Atrial Fibrillation

If you have atrial fibrillation, preventing blood clots is crucial because it reduces the risk of stroke. Here's what you need to know:

Why Blood Thinning Matters

People with atrial fibrillation have a higher risk of stroke due to irregular heartbeats. Blood thinning medications help reduce this risk by making blood less likely to clot.

Types of Blood Thinners

1. New Oral Anticoagulants (NOACs/DOACs):

- These are modern medications that are easier to take because they don't require frequent blood tests like older drugs.

- They are effective at reducing stroke risk by 70 to 80%.

2. Vitamin K Antagonists:

- These traditional medications also thin the blood effectively but require regular blood tests (INR tests) every 3 to 4 weeks to monitor dosage.

- The INR value should ideally be between two and three to ensure proper blood thinning.

Taking Blood Thinners

- Consistency is Key: Whether you're on NOACs or vitamin K antagonists, take your medication daily without skipping doses.

- Long-term Use: Most patients with atrial fibrillation need to take blood thinners long-term to maintain their effectiveness.

Considerations

- Monitoring: Even with NOACs, regular check-ups every 6 to 12 months are necessary to assess overall health and adjust treatment if needed.

- Safety Concerns: If you have a higher risk of bleeding, discuss this with your doctor to find the safest treatment approach.

Stopping Blood Thinners

- Doctor's Guidance: Never stop taking blood thinners on your own. If you need to pause them for a medical procedure, your doctor will advise you on when and how to do so safely.

Conclusion

Taking blood thinners as prescribed significantly reduces your risk of stroke if you have atrial fibrillation. It's important to follow your doctor's advice closely and attend regular check-ups to ensure your treatment plan is effective and safe for your health.

Medications for Atrial Fibrillation

If you have atrial fibrillation, medications play a crucial role in managing your condition. Here's what you should know:

Types of Medications

1. Heart Rate Control Medications:

- These medications help slow down a fast heartbeat that often comes with atrial fibrillation.

- They are simpler medications aimed at keeping your heart rate within a normal range.

2. Rhythm Control Medications:

- These medications are stronger and aim to restore your heart to a normal rhythm, called sinus rhythm.

- They are used for patients who experience severe symptoms and need to return to a regular heart rhythm.

Medications for Heart Rate Control

If you have atrial fibrillation, your doctor may prescribe medications to control your heart rate. These include:

- Beta Blockers: These help reduce the heart rate by blocking certain hormones that speed up the heart.

- Calcium Channel Blockers: They relax the heart muscles and can also help control heart rate.
- Digitalis Preparations: These medicines strengthen the heart's contractions and can help control the heartbeat.

Medications for Rhythm Control

For patients with more severe symptoms, medications for rhythm control may be necessary. These include:

- Class I Antiarrhythmics: These medications work by stabilizing the heart's electrical activity to maintain a normal rhythm.
- Class III Antiarrhythmics: They help control irregular heartbeats by affecting the heart's electrical signals.

Benefits and Considerations

- Benefits: Medications can significantly reduce symptoms of atrial fibrillation.
- Considerations: They may have side effects, and their success in restoring a normal heart rhythm may vary among patients.

Monitoring and Side Effects

- Monitoring: Regularly monitor your pulse rate to ensure it stays within a healthy range (60-100 beats per minute).

- Side Effects: Common side effects may include changes in heart rate. Report any unusual symptoms to your doctor promptly.

Conclusion

Medications are important tools in managing atrial fibrillation. They help control heart rate and rhythm, reducing symptoms and improving your quality of life. Work closely with your doctor to find the right medication and monitor your health effectively. Regular check-ups and communication with your healthcare team are essential for successful treatment.

Pacemakers and Treatment Options for Atrial Fibrillation

If you have atrial fibrillation (AFib), your heart may beat irregularly and sometimes too fast or too slow. Here's what you need to know about treatments:

Pacemaker Requirement

For most people with AFib, their heart beats too fast, causing discomfort and stress. However, a small number of patients experience the opposite: their heart beats too slowly. In these cases, instead of medications, they may need a pacemaker.

Success Rates of Drug Therapy

- Frequency Control: About 70% of patients with AFib use medications to control their heart rate while staying in AFib. This often helps reduce symptoms and improve quality of life.

- Rhythm Control: For about a third of patients, the goal is to return the heart to a normal rhythm (sinus rhythm). Medications are an option, but they are successful only about 30 to 40% of the time. Procedures like catheter ablation are more effective for this group.

Understanding the "Rhythm Pill"

If you're younger and have AFib only occasionally, a "rhythm pill" might be an option. This pill isn't taken every day like regular medication. Instead, it's taken only when AFib occurs, aiming to restore normal heart rhythm quickly.

Conditions for Taking the Rhythm Pill

- Suitability: Your doctor will determine if the rhythm pill is right for you based on your health and the frequency of your AFib episodes.

- Initial Examinations: You'll need tests like a heart ultrasound or CT scan before starting this treatment.

- Medical Supervision: The first time you use the rhythm pill, it should be under your doctor's supervision.

Using the Rhythm Pill Effectively

- Rest and Relaxation: After taking the rhythm pill, it's important to rest for the day. Avoid strenuous activities to give the pill time to work and restore normal heart rhythm.

What to Do If the Rhythm Pill Doesn't Work
- Seek Medical Advice: If the rhythm pill doesn't stop AFib within 8 to 12 hours and you have severe symptoms, contact your doctor promptly. They can discuss other treatment options to manage your condition effectively.

Conclusion
Managing atrial fibrillation involves understanding your heart's needs and finding the right treatment. Whether it's medications, procedures like pacemakers, or innovative options like the rhythm pill, your doctor will guide you towards the best choice for your health and well-being. Regular check-ups and open communication with your healthcare team are key to managing AFib successfully.

Cardioversion for Atrial Fibrillation

If you have atrial fibrillation (AFib), your heart beats irregularly, which can cause discomfort and health concerns. Cardioversion is a medical procedure aimed at restoring your heart to a normal rhythm.

What is Cardioversion and When is it Useful?

Cardioversion is used to switch the heart from atrial fibrillation back to a normal rhythm, known as sinus rhythm. This procedure is not something you can do at home—it must be performed in a hospital or outpatient clinic.

How Cardioversion Works

During cardioversion, you may receive a mild anesthesia to help you sleep. Then, a small electric shock is delivered to your chest to reset your heart rhythm. Alternatively, medications can also be used to achieve the same effect.

Suitability for Patients

Cardioversion is suitable for patients who need rhythm control to manage their AFib. However, it's effective for only about a third to a quarter of AFib patients.

Duration and Effectiveness

In about 90% of cases, cardioversion successfully restores normal heart rhythm almost immediately. However, it does not prevent AFib from returning. Additional treatments like daily medications or catheter ablation may be needed to maintain normal rhythm long-term.

Preparing for Cardioversion

Before undergoing cardioversion, your doctor may recommend a transesophageal echocardiogram (swallowing ultrasound) to check for blood clots in your heart. This is crucial because cardioversion can dislodge clots, leading to a stroke.

- Swallowing Ultrasound: This quick and painless procedure takes 10 to 15 minutes and helps ensure your safety during cardioversion.

Procedure and Follow-Up

The actual cardioversion procedure is brief, usually lasting only a fraction of a second. Its success in restoring normal rhythm can be immediately seen on an ECG (electrocardiogram). After cardioversion, ongoing treatment is necessary to maintain the normal heart rhythm achieved.

Advantages and Risks
Cardioversion is highly effective and has a low risk of complications when performed under proper conditions, such as adequate blood thinning or a clear ultrasound scan.

Patient Responsibilities
- Medication: Continuously take prescribed medications, including blood thinners, even on the day of cardioversion.
- Fasting: Arrive for the procedure on an empty stomach, following fasting instructions from your doctor.
- Medical Information: Inform your healthcare team about any allergies or reactions to medications.

Cardioversion is a valuable treatment option for restoring normal heart rhythm in patients with atrial fibrillation. By understanding the procedure and following your doctor's guidance, you can contribute to a successful outcome and better manage your condition. Regular communication with your healthcare provider is essential for ongoing care and monitoring.

Ablation for Atrial Fibrillation

Ablation is a modern treatment method for atrial fibrillation (AFib), a condition where the heart beats irregularly. This procedure aims to restore and maintain a normal heart rhythm.

What is Ablation?

Ablation involves inserting thin tubes (called catheters) into the heart through the groin. These catheters are used to target and treat specific areas in the heart responsible for causing atrial fibrillation.

Procedure Details

During the procedure, which takes place in a hospital, the catheters are guided to the heart's left atrium where the pulmonary veins are located. These veins carry blood from the lungs to the heart and can trigger atrial fibrillation when they malfunction.

Types of Ablation

There are different types of ablation techniques:

- Radiofrequency Ablation: Uses heat to cauterize (burn) the problematic heart tissue.
- Cryoablation: Involves freezing the abnormal tissue to restore normal heart rhythm.

- Electroporation: A newer method that uses electric shocks to treat atrial fibrillation without heat or cold.

These methods are chosen based on what will work best for each patient's specific condition.

Preparing for Ablation
Before undergoing ablation, several tests are conducted to determine if you are a suitable candidate. These tests include an ultrasound to measure your heart's size and an ECG to record your heart's electrical activity.

During the Procedure
You will receive light anesthesia to make you comfortable during the procedure, which typically lasts between 45 to 90 minutes. Most patients spend one or two nights in the hospital for observation.

After the Procedure
After ablation, it's important to follow these guidelines:
- Continue Blood Thinners: Most AFib patients need to continue taking blood thinners after ablation to prevent blood clots.

- Take it Easy: Avoid strenuous activities like sports or heavy lifting for the first 1 to 2 weeks to allow your body to heal.
- Follow-Up Checks: Attend follow-up appointments to ensure the ablation was successful and to adjust your treatment plan as needed.

Benefits and Risks of Ablation

Ablation has a success rate of up to 80%, which is higher than using medications alone (30-40%). It offers a chance to potentially cure atrial fibrillation and reduce the need for ongoing medication, except for blood thinners.

What Happens After Ablation?

After undergoing catheter ablation for atrial fibrillation, it's important to understand what to expect during the healing process and how to care for yourself.

Recovery Period

You will typically return home the day after the procedure with a small bandage over the entry point in your groin where the catheters were inserted. It's essential to take care of this area to prevent any complications.

Physical Rest
For the first one or two weeks after ablation, it's best to avoid strenuous activities like sports or heavy lifting. Your heart may feel sensitive during this time, and you might occasionally feel heart palpitations. This is normal as your heart heals from the procedure.

Returning to Normal Activities
After a successful procedure, you can gradually resume your normal activities. You may feel ready to return to work within a few days if you're feeling well. Sports and other physical activities can usually be resumed after about 1 to 2 weeks, depending on how you feel.

Follow-Up Care
It's crucial to schedule a follow-up appointment with your doctor a few weeks or months after the procedure. This visit will assess how successful the ablation was in restoring your normal heart rhythm and determine any further steps needed for your care.

Success and Risks
The success rate of catheter ablation for atrial fibrillation can vary. In ideal conditions, it can be as high as 80%, gradually decreasing with

other heart conditions or longer periods of atrial fibrillation. If the first procedure isn't successful, it can be repeated to increase the chances of curing atrial fibrillation.

Potential Side Effects

Modern methods have reduced the occurrence of side effects, but some patients may still experience mild issues like groin bleeding (1-2% of cases). Serious complications, such as heart injuries, are rare.

Conclusion

Catheter ablation aims to improve your quality of life by treating atrial fibrillation effectively. As with any medical procedure, it's essential to discuss with your doctor to fully understand the benefits, risks, and recovery process involved.

By following these guidelines and staying informed, you can manage your recovery effectively and return to enjoying your daily activities.

CHAPTER NINE

Natural Treatments for Atrial Fibrillation

Can Atrial Fibrillation be Reversed Naturally?

Many people newly diagnosed with atrial fibrillation wonder if they can reverse it naturally. Living with this condition, which causes sudden, rapid heartbeats, can greatly affect daily life and cause anxiety. In this chapter, we explore natural treatment options that can significantly improve AFib symptoms through lifestyle changes.

Can You Treat Atrial Fibrillation with Natural Supplements?

When thinking about natural treatments, people often consider over-the-counter supplements and vitamins. However, current research shows that none of these products have proven to effectively reduce AFib symptoms. Omega-3 fish oils and magnesium supplements, commonly used for heart health, have not shown long-term success in treating AFib.

How to Reverse Atrial Fibrillation Naturally – Lifestyle Changes and Commitment

Committing to healthy lifestyle changes is the key to managing AFib symptoms naturally. Research indicates that these changes can lead to long-term success in managing AFib:

- Reduce Medication Dependence: By making consistent lifestyle changes, you may be able to lower the dosage and frequency of conventional AFib medications.

- Avoid Invasive Procedures: Lifestyle changes can also reduce the need for invasive surgeries related to AFib treatment.

- Prolong Positive Health Outcomes: They can enhance the benefits of other AFib treatments you may have undergone.

Lifestyle Changes that Positively Impact AFib Symptoms

Small but significant lifestyle adjustments can make a big difference in managing AFib:

- Avoid Stimulants: Limiting intake of caffeine, chocolate, and energy drinks can help stabilize heart rate and improve AFib symptoms.

- Adjust Your Diet: Including more vegetables, fruits, and lean proteins while reducing trans fats and sugars can benefit overall health and AFib symptoms.

- Stay Hydrated: Drinking enough water helps prevent dehydration, which can stress the body. Cutting back on alcohol can also improve AFib symptoms.

- Stay Active: Engaging in gentle activities like walking, gardening, or yoga supports heart health and reduces stress, which can impact AFib. You don't need intense workouts to see benefits.

These lifestyle changes, when combined with commitment and regular follow-up with your healthcare provider, offer a natural approach to managing atrial fibrillation and improving your quality of life.

CHAPTER TEN

The Future of AFib Treatment

Researching a New Drug for Atrial Fibrillation

A team supported by the German Heart Foundation is investigating a promising new drug that could revolutionize treatment for patients with atrial fibrillation (AFib). This condition causes sudden, irregular heartbeats that leave patients feeling weak, dizzy, and nauseous. But there's hope on the horizon!

According to current research, this new drug swiftly restores normal heart rhythm and is well tolerated by patients. If ongoing research proves successful, it could greatly enhance the treatment of acute AFib in the future, significantly improving the quality of life for those affected.

Effectiveness of the New Drug for Acute AFib

Treating atrial fibrillation with medication is currently limited, but this may change soon. Recently, a team at Heidelberg University

Hospital identified a specific cause behind AFib development: TASK-1 ion channels in the human atrium. These channels play a crucial role in the electrical activity of heart muscle cells in the atria, where AFib originates.

Funded by the German Heart Foundation, the research team discovered that patients with AFib have higher levels of these ion channels compared to those with healthy hearts. This discovery led to the development of a drug that targets and blocks these channels, restoring normal heart rhythm. Initial tests with an approved drug, previously used for another condition, began in 2019 and have shown promising results with good tolerance.

Advantages of the Research Project
This research is unique because the drug specifically targets TASK-1 ion channels found only in the atria. Unlike conventional antiarrhythmic drugs, which affect multiple heart chambers and can lead to long-term side effects, this targeted approach minimizes unwanted effects elsewhere in the body. The drug also acts rapidly, providing relief soon after administration, based on early testing.

The study aims to establish optimal dosages for different patients and evaluate any potential side effects. Participants, hospitalized for acute AFib, receive the drug intravenously and undergo monitoring with long-term ECG for six hours to assess its effectiveness.

RESOURCES

Atrial fibrillation is the most common arrhythmia in humans. It occurs in 2.5 percent of the population. It is important to know that the older you get, the higher your risk of developing atrial fibrillation. ([Mayo Clinic](https://www.mayoclinic.org/diseases-conditions/atrial-fibrillation/symptoms-causes/syc-20350624))

Funding source: The research project is funded by the German Heart Foundation ([Deutsche Herzstiftung](https://www.deutsche-herzstiftung.de/)).